PREMIUM ORGASM

The secret behind every woman's sexual climax unvailed.

By

Dr. Vicente L. Delgado

Introduction

The climax is one of the most extraordinary joys feasible to a creature, yet its hidden components remain ineffectively comprehended. Based on existing written works, **Premium orgasm** presents a clever unthinking model of sexual feeling and climax. In doing as such, it portrays the neurophenomenology of sexual daze and peak, depicts matches in elements among climaxes and seizures, guesses on conceivable transformative beginnings of sex contrasts in orgasmic answering, and proposes roads for future trial and error. Here, a model is presented wherein sexual feeling incites the entrainment of coupling mechanical and neuronal oscillatory frameworks, hence making synchronized useful organizations inside which different good input processes meet synergistically to add to sexual experience. These cycles produce conditions of extending tangible retention and daze, possibly finishing in peak assuming basic edges are outperformed. The centrality of cadenced feeling (and its tweak by remarkable quality) for outperforming these limits recommends manners by which differential orgasmic answering between people — or with various accomplices — may act as an instrument for guaranteeing versatile mate decision. Since the development of musical excitement consolidates legit signs of wellness with prompts connecting with potential for the venture, the differential orgasmic reaction might effectively impact the likelihood of proceeding with sexual experiences with explicit mates.

Table Of Contents

Chapter 1: Sexual Climax (Orgasm)

Chapter 2: Trouble Arriving At Sexual Climax
- Orgasmic Brokenness
- Untimely Discharge
- Vulvodynia
-

Chapter 3: Things To Know About Female Climaxes, And How To Reach Yours

Chapter 1

Sexual climax

What is sexual Climax?

Sexual climax or orgasm is the abrupt release of amassed sexual fervor during the sexual reaction cycle, bringing about a musical, compulsory strong withdrawals in the pelvic locale described by sexual delight. Experienced by guys and females, climaxes are constrained by the compulsory or autonomic sensory system. They are normally connected with compulsory activities, remembering solid fits for numerous regions of the body, an overall euphoric sensation, and, much of the time, body developments and vocalizations. The period after sexual climax (known as the recalcitrant period) is regularly a loosening up encounter, credited to the arrival of the neurohormones oxytocin and prolactin as well as endorphins (or "endogenous morphine").

Human climaxes as a rule result from actual sexual excitement of the penis in guys (commonly going with discharge) and of the clitoris in females. Sexual excitement can be by self-practice (masturbation) or with a sex accomplice (penetrative sex, non-penetrative sex, or another sexual movement).

The well-being impacts encompassing the human climax are assorted. There are numerous physiological reactions during sexual activity, including a casual state made by prolactin, as well as changes in the focal sensory system, for example, a brief lessening in the metabolic movement of enormous pieces of the cerebral cortex while there is no change or expanded metabolic action in the limbic (i.e., "lining") region of the cerebrum. There is likewise a great many sexual dysfunctions, like anorgasmia. These impacts influence social perspectives on a climax, for example, the convictions that climax and the recurrence or consistency of it are either significant or unimportant for fulfillment in a sexual relationship, and hypotheses about the natural and developmental elements of the climax

In a clinical setting, the sexual climax is generally characterized rigorously by the solid compressions required during sexual action, alongside the trademark examples of a shift in perspective rate, circulatory strain, frequent breath rate, and profundity. This is ordered as the abrupt release of collected sexual pressure during the sexual reaction cycle, bringing about cadenced strong constrictions in the pelvic locale. Notwithstanding, meanings of climax differ and there is a feeling that agreement on the most proficient method to reliably group it is missing.

There is some discussion about whether specific kinds of sexual sensations ought to be precisely delegated climaxes, including female climaxes brought about by Sweet spot excitement alone, and the exhibition of expanded or persistent climaxes enduring a few minutes or even 60 minutes. The inquiry is based on the clinical meaning of sexual climax, however, this approach to reviewing sexual climax is simply physiological, while there are additionally mental, endocrinological, and neurological meanings of sexual climax. In these and comparable cases, the sensations experienced are emotional and don't be guaranteed to include the compulsory compressions normal for a sexual climax. Notwithstanding, the sensations in the two genders are very pleasurable and are in many cases felt all through the body, causing a psychological expression that is frequently portrayed as supernatural, and with vasocongestion and related delight similar to that of a full-contractionary climax. For instance, present-day discoveries support qualification among discharge and male climax. Consequently, there are sees on the two sides concerning whether these can be precisely characterized as climaxes.

Climaxes can be accomplished during different exercises, including vaginal, butt-centric, or oral sex, non-penetrative sex, or masturbation. They may likewise be accomplished by the utilization of a sex toy, like an exotic vibrator or a suggestive electrostimulation. Accomplishing climax by feeling the areolas or other erogenous zones is more extraordinary. Numerous climaxes are additionally conceivable, particularly in ladies, however, they are likewise phenomenal. Various climaxes are climaxes that happen within a brief time of each other.

Notwithstanding actual feeling, climax can be accomplished from mental excitement alone, for example, during dreaming (nighttime outflow for guys or females) or by the constrained climax. Climax by mental feeling alone was first detailed among individuals who had spinal line injuries. Albeit sexual capability and sexuality, after spinal string injury is frequently influenced, this injury doesn't deny one of the sexual sentiments like sexual excitement and suggestive longings.

Logical writing centers around the brain science of female climax essentially more than it does on the brain science of male climax, which "seems to mirror the supposition that female climax is mentally more mind-boggling than the male climax," yet "the restricted exact proof accessible proposes that male and female climax might bear a greater number of similitudes than contrasts. In one controlled concentrate by Vance and Wagner (1976), free raters couldn't separate composed portrayals of male versus female climax encounters.

The capability or elements of the human female orgasm have been bantered among analysts. Analysts have a few speculations about the job, if any, of the female climax in the regenerative and hence transformative cycle. The writing began with the contention that the female climax is a result of shared early male ontogeny, where the male climax is a variation. Research has moved to examine and support the sire-decision speculation, which recommends that the female climax has been molded by regular choice to work in the determination of top-notch sires (male guardians) for posterity. In this way, the climax builds the possibility of imagining guys of high hereditary quality. Research by Randy Thornhill (1995) recommended that female climax is more continuous during intercourse with a male band together with low fluctuating unevenness.

Guys
Inconstancies

In men, the most well-known approach to accomplishing climax is by the actual sexual excitement of the penis. This is generally joined by discharge, yet it is conceivable, however likewise intriguing, for men to climax without discharge (known as a "dry climax"). Juvenile young men have dry climaxes. Dry climaxes can likewise happen because of retrograde discharge, or hypogonadism. Men may likewise discharge without arriving at the climax, which is known as an orgasmic discharge.

Customary view

The customary perspective on male climax is that there are two phases: discharge going with a climax, immediately followed by a stubborn period. The hard-headed period is the recuperation stage after the climax during which it is physiologically beyond the realm of possibilities for a man to have extra climaxes. In 1966, Bosses and Johnson distributed urgent examinations about the periods of sexual feeling. Their work included ladies and men, and, not at all like Alfred Kinsey in 1948 and 1953, attempted to decide the physiological stages when climax.

Experts and that's what johnson contended, in the principal stage, "embellishment organs contract and the male can feel the discharge coming; a few seconds after the fact the discharge happens, which the man can't compel, delay, or in any capacity control" and that, in the subsequent stage, "the male feels pleasurable constrictions during discharge, detailing more prominent delight attached to a more prominent volume of discharge". That's what they detailed, in contrast to females, "for the man the goal stage incorporates a superimposed recalcitrant period" and added that "numerous guys beneath the age of 30, yet generally few from there on, can discharge habitually and are likely to, without a doubt, exceptionally short headstrong periods during the goal stage". Experts and Johnson compared male climax and discharge and kept up with the need for a hard-headed period between climaxes.

Ensuing and numerous climaxes

There has been a minimal logical investigation of various climaxes in men. Dunn and Trost characterized male various climaxes as "at least two climaxes regardless of discharge and without, or with, truth be told, exceptionally restricted, de-distension (loss of erection) during very much the same sexual experience". Albeit, because of the recalcitrant period, it is uncommon for men to accomplish numerous climaxes, a few men have revealed having various, continuous climaxes, especially without discharge. There may not be a conspicuous stubborn period, and the last climax might cause an unmanageable period. Different climaxes are more regularly detailed in extremely young fellows than in more established men. In more youthful men, the unmanageable period may just last a couple of moments, however, last over an hour in more established men.

An expanded mixture of the chemical oxytocin during discharge is accepted to be mostly liable for the unmanageable period, and the sum by which oxytocin is expanded may influence the length of every recalcitrant period. A logical report to effectively record regular, completely ejaculatory, various climaxes in a grown-up man was led at Rutgers College in 1995. During the review, six completely ejaculatory climaxes were knowledgeable about 36 minutes, with no evident obstinate period.

Females

Orgasmic elements and changeabilities

In ladies, the most well-known method for accomplishing climax is by a direct sexual feeling of the clitoris (meaning steady manual, oral, or another concentrated grinding against the outer pieces of the clitoris). General insights show that 70-80% of ladies require direct clitoral feeling to accomplish climax, albeit roundabout clitoral excitement (for instance, through vaginal infiltration) may likewise be adequate. The Mayo Facility expressed, "Climaxes change in force, and ladies fluctuate in the recurrence of their climaxes and how much excitement is important to set off a climax." Clitoral climaxes are simpler to accomplish because the glans of the clitoris, or clitoris, all in all, has above 8,000 tactile sensitive spots, which is as many (or more at times) sensitive spots as are available in the human penis or glans penis. As the clitoris is homologous to the penis, it is the same in its ability to get sexual excitement.

Chapter 2

Trouble arriving at sexual climax

Orgasmic brokenness

Orgasmic brokenness is a condition that happens when somebody experiences issues arriving at the climax. This trouble happens in any event when they're physically stirred and there's adequate sexual feeling. At the point when this condition happens in ladies, it's known as female orgasmic brokenness. Men can likewise encounter orgasmic brokenness, yet this is substantially less normal.

Climaxes are extreme sensations of delivery during sexual excitement. They can shift in power, length, and recurrence. Climaxes can happen with minimal sexual feeling, yet now and again significantly more excitement is vital.

Numerous ladies experience issues arriving at the climax with an accomplice, even after more than adequate sexual excitement. Studies recommend orgasmic brokenness influences 11 to 41 percent of trusted Wellspring of ladies.

Orgasmic brokenness is otherwise called anorgasmia or female orgasmic problem.

What causes orgasmic brokenness?

It very well may be challenging to decide the hidden reason for orgasmic brokenness. Ladies might experience issues arriving at climax due to physical, close-to-home, or mental elements. Contributing elements could include:

- more seasoned age
- ailments, like diabetes
- a background marked by gynecological medical procedures, like a hysterectomy
- the utilization of specific meds, especially particular serotonin reuptake inhibitors (SSRIs) for gloom
- social or strict convictions
- timidity
- responsibility about appreciating sexual action
- history of sexual maltreatment

- emotional wellness conditions, like gloom or uneasiness
- stress
- unfortunate confidence
- relationship issues, like irritating contentions or absence of trust

Once in a while, a blend of these variables can make accomplishing a climax troublesome. The powerlessness to climax can prompt misery, which might make it much harder to accomplish climax from here on out.

What are the side effects of orgasmic brokenness?

The fundamental side effect of orgasmic brokenness is the failure to accomplish a sexual peak. Different side effects incorporate having uninspiring climaxes and taking more time than typical to arrive at a peak. Ladies with orgasmic brokenness might experience issues accomplishing climax during sex or masturbation.

There are four sorts of orgasmic brokenness:

Essential anorgasmia: A condition wherein you've never had a climax.

Optional anorgasmia: Trouble arriving at the climax, even though you've had one preceding.

Situational anorgasmia: The most well-known kind of orgasmic brokenness. It happens when you can climax during explicit circumstances, for example, during oral sex or masturbation.

General anorgasmia: A failure to accomplish climax for any reason, in any event, when you're exceptionally stirred and sexual feeling is adequate.

How is orgasmic brokenness analyzed?

Assuming you assume you have orgasmic brokenness, you ought to plan a meeting with your PCP. Your PCP will want to analyze your condition and give a legitimate treatment plan. Finding support from your primary care physician is the most effective way to guarantee that you can completely appreciate sexual action once more.

During your arrangement, your primary care physician will pose inquiries about your sexual history and carry out an actual assessment. Your reactions and test results can uncover any fundamental reasons for orgasmic brokenness and can assist with distinguishing different elements that might be adding to your condition.

Your primary care physician might allude you to a gynecologist for a subsequent test. A gynecologist can suggest further medicines for orgasmic brokenness.

How is orgasmic brokenness treated?

Treatment for orgasmic brokenness relies upon the reason for the condition. You might have to:

- treat any hidden ailments
- switch stimulant meds
- have mental social treatment (CBT) or sex treatment
- increment clitoral feeling during masturbation and sex

Couples directing is another famous treatment choice. An instructor will assist you and your cooperation with managing any conflicts or clashes you might have. This can determine the issues that are happening both in the relationship and in the room.

At times, estrogen chemical treatment might be utilized. Estrogen can assist with expanding sexual craving or how much bloodstream to the privates for elevated responsiveness. Estrogen chemical treatment might include taking a pill, wearing a fix, or applying a gel to the privates. Testosterone treatment is another choice. Notwithstanding, the U.S. Food and Medication Organization (FDA) hasn't supported it for treating orgasmic brokenness in ladies.

Some over-the-counter (OTC) items and wholesome enhancements may likewise assist ladies with orgasmic brokenness. Excitement oils, like Zestra, warm the clitoris and increment feeling. These oils might be gainful to use during sex and masturbation. Ensure you talk with your PCP before utilizing any OTC items or meds. They might cause an unfavorably susceptible response or obstruct different drugs you're taking.

What's the standpoint for individuals with orgasmic brokenness?

The powerlessness to climax can be disappointing and may affect your relationship. In any case, you might have the option to arrive at peak with legitimate treatment. It's vital to know that you're in good company. Numerous ladies manage orgasmic brokenness eventually in their lives.

Assuming you have orgasmic brokenness, you might view treatment as especially supportive. Part of individual or couples treatment centers around how you view sex. Meeting with a specialist can assist you and your band together with diving deeper into another's sexual requirements and wants. It will likewise address any relationship issues or regular stressors that might be adding to your failure to climax. Settling these fundamental causes can assist you with arriving at a climax from now on.

Untimely discharge

Discharge (otherwise known as "cumming") is when semen sprays out of the launch of the urethra in your penis, normally during sex or masturbation. Untimely discharge is the point at which you discharge (cum) before you need to — normally before your accomplice has a climax.

Untimely discharge is normal, particularly for more youthful individuals. Essentially nothing remains to be stressed over on the off chance that it happens occasionally. However, it very well may be viewed as a clinical issue on the off chance that it happens the greater part of the times you attempt to have intercourse.

What causes untimely discharge?

No one realizes without a doubt what causes untimely discharge, yet it's most probable mental or profound. Untimely discharge isn't brought about by illnesses, contaminations, or issues with your sensory system.

Are there untimely discharge medicines?

There are various medicines for untimely discharge. Your attendant or specialist can assist you with concluding which treatment might turn out best for you.

Treatment choices include:

- Guiding or treatment, including things like sex treatment or stress decrease
- Physician endorsed medication that can protract the time before climax

- Restricting your utilization of liquor and different medications
- Unwinding and breathing activities
- Coordinated masturbation practices that incorporate easing back and halting to assist you with figuring out how to remain hard (erect) without discharging
- Stroking off with an accomplice

Rehearsing sex with an accomplice where you "respite and crush". This implies that you quit having intercourse when you feel near cumming and press behind the tip of your penis until the inclination disappears. Then you begin having intercourse once more.

Vulvodynia

Vulvodynia is a condition when you have torment in your vulva (Also known as vulvar agony) that isn't from a disease or other clinical issue, and it goes on for quite a long time or more.

Vulvodynia side effects incorporate torment and disturbance like consuming, stinging, crudeness, hurting, irritation, pounding, and expanding. This might influence your entire vulva or just a single explicit region. If your vulvar aggravation is in the tissue at the launch of your vagina (called the vestibule), you might have a kind of vulvodynia called vestibulodynia, otherwise called vulvar vestibulitis.

You can have vulvodynia side effects constantly, or they can go back and forth. Side effects can happen haphazardly or just when something contacts your vulva or goes inside your vagina. Things that put a squeeze on your vulva — like sex, utilizing a tampon, getting a pelvic test, wearing tight jeans, or sitting for quite a while — can set off vulvodynia side effects or exacerbate them.

What causes vulvodynia?

Vulvodynia frequently doesn't have a particular reason. It probably has loads of various causes cooperating, including things like:

- Nerve disturbance or nerve harm in your vulva
- Irritation (expanding) in your vulva
- A few hereditary issues, such as ongoing torment or issues battling contaminations
- Issues with your pelvic floor muscles

- Responses to specific contaminations
- Food responsive qualities
- Conditions that influence the muscles or bones close to your vulva
- Sexual maltreatment or injury from before

Are there vulvodynia medicines?

On the off chance that you have vulvar torment, make a meeting with a specialist or medical caretaker, similar to the ones at your neighborhood Arranged Life as a parent wellbeing focus. They'll give you a test and ask you inquiries about your side effects and clinical history to attempt to assist with sorting out what's causing your vulvar aggravation. The medical caretaker or specialist might take an example of your vaginal release, and contact portions of your vulva with a q-tip to see where you have torment and how severely it harms. At times they may likewise do a biopsy of a limited quantity of skin from the area.

There are bunches of medicines for vulvodynia, yet all the same, everybody's unique. So there's not one treatment that works for everybody. You could have to attempt more than one treatment, and it can require a couple of months before you begin to feel improved.

Vulvodynia treatment can include:
- Medications like sedatives (creams that insensible aggravation), antidepressants, hostile to seizure meds, and chemical creams.
- Active recuperation assists with loosening up your pelvic floor tissues or fortifying your pelvic muscles (the muscles around your vulva/vagina).
- Trigger point treatment that utilizations knead or potentially shots that have a blend of pain relievers and steroids to treat a little region where your muscles are tight.
- Different shots like a nerve block (pain relievers for the nerves that cause you to feel torment) or botox (an injection of medication that loosens up your pelvic floor muscles).
- Utilizing ultrasound or electrical feeling to assist with facilitating torment.

Now and again, medical procedures to eliminate tissue from the vestibule (the region close to your vaginal opening), assuming that is the main spot you have torment and different therapies haven't worked. Managing vulvodynia can be hard both truly and inwardly. It might assist with seeking psychological wellness guidance like mental social treatment or sexual treatment, which can assist you with managing the profound impacts of persistent torment and the effect vulvodynia may have on your sexual coexistence and connections.

Chapter 3

Things To Know About Female Climaxes, And How To Reach Yours

Is this a specific sort of climax?

No, "female climax" is a widely inclusive term for a climax connected with female genitalia.

It very well may be clitoral, vaginal, even cervical — or a blend of every one of the three. All things considered, your genitalia isn't your main choice about accomplishing the large O.

Peruse on for tips on where to contact, how to move, why it works, and the sky is the limit from there.

It very well may be a clitoral climax

Immediate or circuitous excitement of the clitoris can prompt a clitoral climax. At the point when you get your rub on perfectly, you'll feel the sensation work in your pleasure bud and pinnacle.

Attempt this

Your fingers, palm, or a little vibrator can all assist you with having a clitoral climax.

Ensure your clitoris is wet and start tenderly focusing on a side-to-side or all-over movement.

As it feels far better, apply quicker and harder tension in a dull movement.

At the point when you feel your pleasure heighten, apply considerably more strain to the movement to take yourself past the brink.

It very well may be a vaginal climax

Albeit hardly any individuals can peak with vaginal feeling alone, it sure can fun attempt!

Assuming you're ready to get it going, plan for an extraordinary peak that can be felt somewhere inside your body.

The front vaginal wall is likewise home to the foremost fornix, or A-spot.

More established research recommends that invigorating the A-spot can bring about serious grease and even climax.

Attempt this

Fingers or a sex toy ought to get the job done. Since the joy comes from the vaginal walls, you'll need to explore different avenues regarding width. Do this by embedding an additional finger or two into the vagina, or attempt a sex play with some additional bigness.

To animate the A-spot, center the tension around the front mass of the vagina while sliding your fingers or toy in and out. Stay with the tension and movement that feels the best, and let the joy mount.

It very well may be a cervical climax

Cervical excitement can prompt a full-body climax that can send rushes of shivery delight from your head to your toes.

Furthermore, this is a climax that can continue to give, enduring a long time for some.

Your cervix is the lower end of your uterus, so arriving at it implies diving in deep.

Attempt this

Being loose and stimulated is vital to accomplishing a cervical climax. Utilize your creative mind, rub your clitoris, or let your accomplice work some foreplay enchantment.

The from the rear position considers profound infiltration, so take a stab at being down on the ground with a penetrative toy or accomplice.

Get going sluggish, steadily working your direction more profoundly until you find a profundity that feels quite a bit better, and keep at it so the joy can fabricate.

Or on the other hand a blend of all the abovementioned

A combo climax can be accomplished by pleasuring your vagina and clitoris all the while.

The outcome: a strong peak that you can feel all around.

Make certain to supersize your combo by including a few other erogenous zones along with everything else.

Attempt this

Utilize both your hands to twofold your pleasure, or consolidate fingers and sex toys. Bunny vibrators, for instance, can animate the clitoris and vagina simultaneously and are ideal for dominating the combo climax.

Utilize equal rhythms while playing with your clitoris and vagina, or change everything around with quick clitoral activity and slow vaginal entrance.

In any case, you can O from other feelings, as well

The private parts are marvelous, however, they're not your main choice. Your body is brimming with erogenous zones with orgasmic potential.

Areola

Your areolas are brimming with sensitive spots that can feel quite great when played with.

As indicated by a recent report, when invigorated, your areolas set your genital tactile cortex on fire. This is the very region of the cerebrum that lights up during vaginal or clitoral feeling.

Areola climaxes are said to surprise you, then detonate in rushes of full-body delight. Certainly!

Attempt this: Utilization your hands to stroke and crush your bosoms and different pieces of your body, staying away from the areolas right away.

Continue toward prodding your areola by following it with your fingertips until you're truly turned on, then, at that point, show your areolas a little love by scouring and squeezing them until you arrive at the greatest joy.

Butt-centric

You don't have to have a prostate to have a butt-centric climax. Butt-centric play can be pleasurable for anybody assuming you have sufficient lube and take as much time as is needed.

You can by implication invigorate erogenous zones inside the vagina utilizing a finger or sex toy.

Attempt this: Apply more than adequate lube with your fingers and back rub it around your rear end. This won't simply lube you up — it'll likewise assist with preparing you for butt-centric play.

Rub the outside and within the opening, then leisurely and delicately embed your sex toy or finger into your rear end. Attempt a delicate in and out movement, then, at that point, start to move in a roundabout movement. Switch back and forth between the two and quit slacking as your pleasure fabricates.

Erogenous zones

Your body truly is a wonderland. The neck, ears, and lower back, for instance, are wealthy in sexually charged sensitive spots asking to be contacted.

We can't say precisely what parts of your body will push you to the edge, yet we can let you know that everybody has erogenous zones, and finding them is most certainly worth the work.

Attempt this: Take a quill or smooth scarf and use it to track down your body's most delicate regions.

Get bare and unwind so you can zero in on each shiver. Observe these spots, and have a go at trying different things with various sensations, such as crushing or squeezing.

Careful discipline brings about promising results, so joy these regions and keep at it to find out how far you can turn out.

Where does the Sweet spot come in?
The Sweet spot is a region along the front mass of your vagina. For certain individuals, it can deliver an exceptionally extraordinary and extremely wet climax when invigorated.
Your fingers or a bent Sweet spot vibrator are the most ideal way to raise a ruckus around town. Crouching will give you the best point.

Attempt this: Squat with the rear of your thighs near or contacting your heels, and addition your fingers or toy into your vagina. Twist your fingers up toward your stomach button and move them in a "come here" movement.
Assuming you end up finding a region that feels better, continue onward — regardless of whether you feel like you need to pee — and partake in the full-body discharge.

What occurs in the body when you climax? Does this rely upon the kind?
Each body is unique, as are its climaxes. Some are more extreme. Some last longer. Some are wetter.

What genuinely occurs during the climax is:

- Your vagina and uterus contract quickly.
- You experience compulsory muscle compressions in different parts, similar to your mid-region and feet.
- Your pulse and breathing revive.
- Your pulse increments.
- You might feel an unexpected help of sexual pressure, or even discharge.

What makes a female climax not the same as a male climax?

It could be amazing, however, they're not exactly unique.

Both include expanded blood stream to the private parts, quicker breathing and pulse, and muscle withdrawals.

Where they regularly contrast is in length and recuperation — otherwise called radiance.

The female climax may likewise endure longer, going from 13 to 51 seconds by and large, while the male climax frequently goes from 10 to 30 seconds.

Individuals with a vagina can regularly have more climaxes whenever invigorated once more.

Individuals with a penis commonly have a headstrong stage. Climaxes are absurd during this period, which can endure from minutes to days.

Individuals with a clitoris may likewise go through a comparable stage. A recent report including 174 college understudies found that 96% of female members experienced touchiness in the clitoris following climax.

Keep in mind, the scope of the hard-headed stage changes from one individual to another. Your own experience is extraordinary to you.

Then there's discharge. For an individual with a penis, compressions force semen into the urethra and out of the penis. What's more, talking about discharge…

Is female discharge a thing?

Indeed! What's more, it's a genuinely normal thing.

A 2013 examination survey of female discharge tracked down that more than 10 to 54 percent trusted Wellspring of members experienced discharge during the climax.

Discharge happens when liquid is ousted from your urethral opening during climax or sexual excitement. The discharge is a thick, whitish liquid that looks like watered-down milk. It contains a portion of similar parts to semen.

What's the climax hole?
The climax hole alludes to the hole between the quantity of male and female climaxes in hetero sex, where those with female genitalia are getting the more limited finish of the stick.
A recent report on climaxes in hetero lovebird couples found that 87% of spouses and just 49% of wives detailed reliably encountering climaxes during sexual action.

Why the hole? Scientists don't be aware without a doubt. Some contend it very well may be organic, while others fault social and cultural points of view and an absence of training with regards to joy.
I don't think I've climaxed previously, yet I need to — what else is there to do?

If you have a clitoris or a vagina, you realize that genuine climaxes can be not the same as what they show on television.

The principal thing you ought to do is ease the heat off so you can have a ball.

Here it truly is more about the excursion than the objective.

All things being equal, carve out an opportunity to get to know your body and focus on how it feels.

You might find it accommodating to:

- get settled someplace you won't be interfered with or diverted, as in your bed or the shower
- have a go at perusing a suggestive story or involving your creative mind to get yourself in that frame of mind
- rub the plump region over your clitoris and the external and inward lips of your vulva until you start to get wet, perhaps additionally utilizing lube
- begin scouring your clitoris once again with the hood and track down a mood that feels better

- rub quicker and harder, speeding up and strain to strengthen the inclination, and keep at it until you climax

If you don't climax, you can constantly attempt once more. Attempting new things is the most effective way to sort out what turns you on and how to climax.

Vibrator On Her Clit

Utilizing a vibrator on her clit is like scouring her clit with the tip of your finger. Here are a few things you can do with the vibrator on her clit…

- You can drive the tip of it into a specific side of her clit.
- You can rub it over and back on her clit.
- You can focus on it in a circle around her clit gradually/quickly.
- Each lady has methods that she likes. Some need a vibrator-held setup. My recommendation is to try different things with various methods to find which ones she partakes in the most.

Clitoral Hood - A few ladies have an excessively delicate clit. Thus, you might have to involve her clitoral hood as support.

So assuming your accomplice has an excessively delicate clit, rather than straightforwardly contacting it with the vibrator, press it against her clitoral hood.

For particularly touchy ladies, you could have better karma utilizing a vibrator when she's wearing clothing or even jeans.

Sweet Spot Concentration

Zeroing in it on her Sweet Spot is the principal thing that comes to a great many people while utilizing a dildo on their accomplice. Doing this is a basic instance of calculating the dildo so that tension is concerned with her Sweet Spot with each stroke as you are pushing it in and out. Notwithstanding, you could need a dildo with a bend or shaped head explicitly for "G-spotting."

The point and strain that works best will rely upon your accomplice, so criticism is indispensable here. You'll likewise have to explore different avenues regarding quick or slow stroking, yet generally speaking, quicker stroking will give you more feeling. To make her come yet she wants an extreme Sweet spot feeling, a hard glass or even metal dildo could very well get the job done.

Try not to feel that you want a harder erection since she loves glass. She'll in any case like your rooster.

DILDOS

Dildos are the very same as your penis, isn't that so? Also, you can do the same things with them that your penis does, correct?

As a matter of fact, no. On the two counts.

There are both more and less you can do with a dildo, and I'll make sense of why underneath. We'll begin for certain extremely manageable things you ought to give a shot with your young lady and a dildo; then, at that point, we'll get to the tomfoolery stuff.

The primary thing is picking a decent one. Excessively huge and it will be excruciating for your accomplice. Excessively little and she won't feel anything. Think about something regarding the size of your penis assuming she's content with that.

Next is getting the "solidness" right. You can pick a glass or hard plastic dildo, which is fine, however, a few ladies might view this as excessively unbending. Similarly, you can purchase a dildo that is too delicate and twists and flexes excessively. There are a lot of different things to sort out as well. Reasonable looking or oddity formed? Smooth or finished?

As usual, conversing with your young lady is vital here to sort out what's best for both of you and what will make her come.

The Significance of Lube

Many individuals skip lube while utilizing sex toys or in any event, during intercourse. You could feel that you may not have to utilize it. Assuming that your young lady is turned on by you, she'll get wet. She could try and be irritated at the thought, yet here's the reality:

- Lube encourages sex for all interested parties.
- The entrance is more straightforward.
- You can go longer without uneasiness, thus can she.

You can try different things by embedding bigger toys. Also, lube can forestall microtears in her vagina that make her defenseless to contaminations.

You probably won't understand that 30% of ladies experience torment with sex. What's more, when they discuss sex, ladies frequently insinuate sex that doesn't do any harm, rather than discussing sex that feels better or prompts climax.

Honestly, needing to utilize lube doesn't mean she's not turned on. A lady's regular grease changes, and you can never have an excess of lube.

Assuming she's rarely wet, you could have to accomplish other things to turn her on.

Lube is most certainly an unquestionable necessity with butt-centric sex or while utilizing toys anally because the rear end doesn't self-grease up by any means.

Picking lube will make your young lady more agreeable, and that builds the chances you can give her a climax. So go after that bottle while you're snatching a toy or a condom.

JUICING

There is a whole classification of dildos known as 'juicers.' They accompany wrenches, and you turn them around after they're embedded. Most dildos will work with this movement for however long there is not a sharp point that may be awkward.

Before you do embed the dildo and begin turning it, you should are involving a ton of lube to forestall over-the-top grating in a similar spot. Similarly significant is trying to begin gradually on the off chance that it's her most memorable time as well as getting criticism from her on what she appreciates (or hates!).

Jucing is one of those strategies that a few ladies love, yet others could do without it to such an extent.

Remember to get her very horny before you enter her. It'll assist her with appreciating things all the more so you can make her climax.